THIRD EDITION

Breast Cancer:
Myths & Facts

What you need to know

S. EVA SINGLETARY, MD, FACS
Professor of Surgical Oncology
The University of Texas
M. D. Anderson Cancer Center

ALICE F. JUDKINS, RN, MS
Advanced Practice Nurse, Breast Specialist

Text illustrations
by Susan M. Rostan, MFA, EdD

Library of Congress Catalog Card Number 2004-109344

ISBN 1-891483-31-5

Single copies of this book are available at $10.95 each. For information on bulk quantities, contact the publisher, CMP Healthcare Media, Oncology Publishing Group, 600 Community Drive, Manhasset, NY 11030. Telephone: (212) 600-3192.

Printed in the U.S.A.

CMP
United Business Media

Publishers of :
ONCOLOGY
Oncology News International
Cancer Management:
A Multidisciplinary Approach
www.CancerNetwork.com

About the Authors

S. Eva Singletary, MD, is Professor of Surgical Oncology at The University of Texas M. D. Anderson Cancer Center in Houston, Texas. She devotes 100% of her clinical practice to breast cancer patient care in the Nellie B. Connally Multidisciplinary Breast Center. Dr. Singletary received her MD degree in 1977, from the Medical University of South Carolina, Charleston. After a general surgical residency at Shands Teaching Hospital and the University of Florida, Gainesville, she completed a surgical oncology fellowship at The University of Texas M.D. Anderson Cancer Center. She joined The University of Texas faculty in 1985 and received the M. D. Anderson Faculty Achievement Award for Patient Care in 1991. She has served on the President's Cancer Panel Special Commission on Breast Cancer from 1992 to 1994. Dr. Singletary currently serves as chair of the American Joint Committee on Cancer Breast Task Force, and is President of the Society of Surgical Oncology.

Alice F. Judkins, RN, MS, is an Advanced Practice Nurse and Breast Specialist. She received her RN degree in 1960 from Ball State University, Muncie, Indiana. In 1975, after working in a variety of nursing positions from Tasmania, Australia, to Honolulu, Hawaii, Ms. Judkins became Coordinator of the Nurse Practitioner Training Program and Continuing Medical Education Programs for Planned Parenthood of Southeast Texas. She joined The University of Texas M. D. Anderson Cancer Center in 1976 as a Clinical Cancer Detection Specialist and Coordinator of the Breast Module in the University's Cancer Prevention and Detection Program. She began the Long Term Breast Evaluation Clinic in the Department of Surgical Oncology in 1991. Ms. Judkins earned a BA in Health Administration from Ottawa University, Kansas City, Kansas, and an MS from Columbia Pacific University, San Rafael, California. She is the 1996 recipient of the Ethel Fleming Arseneaux Outstanding Nurse Oncologist Award. Ms. Judkins is the recipient of an endowed lectureship series "Leading the Research Revolution in Women's Cancer Care."

Lymph Nodes: Small structures located throughout the body that filter out and destroy bacteria and toxic substances. The lymph nodes are connected by a system of vessels called lymphatics. The lymph nodes can collect cancer cells that travel through the lymphatics.

Lymphedema: Swelling of the arm and/or hand caused by buildup of lymph after an axillary lymph node dissection.

Malignant: Cancerous.

Mammogram: A picture of a breast made using X-rays.

Mammography: The use of X-rays to make pictures of a breast.

Medical Oncologist: A doctor who uses drugs and hormones to treat cancer.

Menopause: The time in a woman's life when the ovaries stop producing the hormones estrogen and progesterone. One of the many symptoms of menopause is the cessation of monthly periods.

Metastasis: The spread of cancer from one part of the body to another. When a cancer spreads to another site, it is said to metastasize.

Modified Radical Mastectomy: Surgery to remove the entire breast (including the nipple) and the axillary lymph nodes. Sometimes called total mastectomy with axillary lymph node dissection.

Myocutaneous Flap: Skin, muscle, and other tissue surgically moved from one part of the body to another to reconstruct a structure (such as a breast) removed for cancer treatment or other reasons.

Needle Localization Biopsy: Biopsy using X-rays and a needle to locate the tissue to be removed. The radiologist takes an X-ray of the breast and places a thin needle in the center of the suspicious area. The surgeon then removes the needle and surrounding tissue. The tissue is examined under a microscope to see if cancer cells are present.

Neoadjuvant Therapy: Chemotherapy given before surgery to shrink a cancer.

Noninvasive: Self-contained; not growing into or destroying healthy tissue. Tumors can be either invasive or noninvasive. Sometimes both types of cells will be present.

Papilloma: A tiny wart-like growth in a breast duct. Papillomas are the most common cause of an amber or bloody nipple discharge.

Pathologist: A doctor who identifies diseases by studying tissue or cells under a microscope.

Prognosis: A prediction about the possible outcome of a disease.

Prosthesis: An artificial replacement for a missing body part. Many women who have had a modified radical or total mastectomy choose to wear a breast prosthesis.

Radiation Oncologist: A doctor who uses radiation to treat cancer or its symptoms.

Radiation Therapy: Treatment using high-energy rays to destroy cancer cells.

Radiologist: A doctor who uses X-rays, ultrasound, and other scans to aid in diagnosis.

Reconstructive Surgery: Surgery to rebuild the shape of the breast.

Recurrence: Reappearance of a cancer. There are three kinds of recurrences: local—at the original site; regional—near the original site; and distant—at another site.

Sentinel Node Biopsy: A simple procedure done to determine the presence of cancer cells in the sentinel nodes, the first nodes likely to be affected if cancer has spread from the breast.

Segmental Mastectomy: Surgery to remove the tumor and a small amount of surrounding breast tissue. Sometimes an axillary lymph node dissection is performed at the same time. Also called partial mastectomy or lumpectomy.

Stage: The extent of the cancer. For breast cancer, the stage is determined by the size of the primary tumor and the presence or absence of cancer cells in lymph nodes and at other body sites.

Surgical Oncologist: A surgeon who specializes in treating cancer.

Total Mastectomy: Surgery to remove the entire breast (including the nipple) but not the axillary lymph nodes.

Tumor: An abnormal growth of cells. A tumor can be either benign or malignant.

Ultrasonography: The use of sound waves to confirm the presence or absence of a mass and to tell the difference between solid tumors and cysts. Also called ultrasound or sonography.

X-ray: A type of radiation. Low doses of X-rays are used to diagnose disease; high doses of X-rays are used to treat cancer. The term is frequently used to refer to the picture created with X-rays.

য়

Contents

Contents *continued*

Introduction

Breast cancer! A diagnosis of breast cancer brings on confusion, uncertainty, fear, and unsolicited advice and can make a woman feel she is losing control of her life. One way a woman may regain control is to help make decisions about her treatment. To do this, she needs accurate information about treatment options and possible outcomes—not the old wives' tales passed on by well-meaning but misguided acquaintances.

We realize that women with breast cancer are asked to make treatment decisions quickly during a period of personal crisis. We have attempted to provide the information you need to work with your doctor to identify treatment goals and weigh the benefits, risks, consequences, and possible outcomes of various treatments. Although this booklet is not a comprehensive guide to treatment options, it does provide essential information to help you make critical decisions about the treatments your doctor describes.

Unfortunately, myths and misconceptions about breast cancer are common and can cause a woman unnecessary fear and confusion. We have identified the most common myths about breast cancer and given you the facts about the disease.

We consider this a handbook that can be carried in a purse or briefcase and read while sitting in a doctor's office or awaiting test results. You can read the booklet from beginning to end or go directly to a particular topic in which you are interested. Words in italics are defined in the Glossary.

Throughout the booklet, you will find quotes from former breast cancer patients. The women describe in their own words their experiences and feelings during and after treatment. We are indebted to these women for their openness and willingness to help others affected by this disease.

What Is Breast Cancer?

Cells in the body normally divide at a steady, even pace. New cells are formed to take the place of old or injured cells. Sometimes, however, when cells divide and multiply rapidly, they form a lump, also called a *tumor*. Tumors can be either *benign* or *malignant*.

Benign tumors are not cancer. They are made up of normal-looking cells. Cells from benign tumors do not invade surrounding tissue or spread to other parts of the body.

Malignant tumors are cancer. They are made up of abnormal-looking cells (Figure 1). Cells from malignant tumors can invade surrounding tissue. They can also break off from the main tumor and spread to other parts of the body by traveling through blood or lymph vessels. The spread of the cancer cells is called *metastasis*.

Myth

All breast cancers occur in the same structures of the breast.

Fact

The majority of breast cancers occur in the ducts of the breast, which connect the milk-producing glands to the nipple. However, some breast cancers occur in the lobules, the milk-producing glands of the breast.

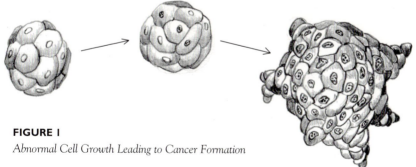

FIGURE 1
Abnormal Cell Growth Leading to Cancer Formation

When a malignant tumor originates in the breast, it is called breast cancer. If this cancer spreads to other parts of the body, it is still called breast cancer. For example, if breast cancer spreads to the lungs, it is called "metastatic breast cancer of the lung" instead of "lung cancer."

The most common site of breast cancer metastasis

4

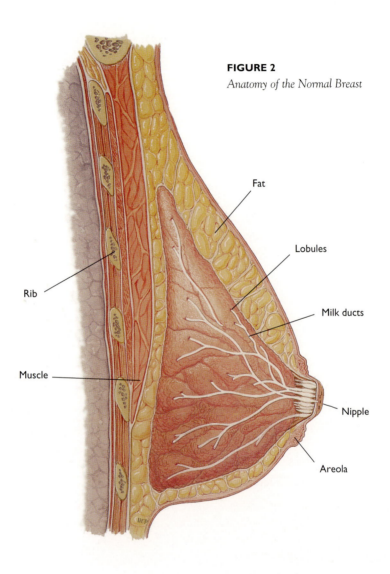

FIGURE 2

Anatomy of the Normal Breast

Fat

Lobules

Milk ducts

Rib

Nipple

Muscle

Areola

Illustration by Harriet Phillips

is the *lymph nodes;* other common sites are the lungs, bones, liver, and brain.

Not all breast cancers are alike. They are not all composed of the same type of abnormal cell. Breast cancers also differ in their location within the breast. Figure 2 shows the anatomy of the normal breast. Most breast cancers arise in the milk ducts and are called *ductal carcinomas.* A small percentage of breast cancers arise in the *lobules* and are called *lobular carcinomas.*

When the cancer is confined within the ducts or lobules, it is called *noninvasive* or in situ cancer. When the cancer has grown into surrounding tissue or spread to other parts of the body, it is called *invasive* cancer.

Breast cancers also differ in their *stage.* Stage is the term used to describe the extent of a cancer. For a breast cancer, the stage is determined by the size of the primary tumor and the presence or absence of cancer cells in lymph nodes and at other body sites.

Myth

All breast cancers are composed of the same type of abnormal cells.

Fact

There are many types of breast cancer, and each is composed of a different type of abnormal cell.

ৰ

What Causes Breast Cancer?

A woman has little or no risk of breast cancer if she has no family history of breast cancer.

More than 75% of women with breast cancer have no family history of the disease. Simply being female puts all women at risk.

Estrogens cause breast cancer.

Recent data have shown that a combination of estrogen and progesterone (HRT) taken by women after menopause may increase the risk of breast cancer if associated with prolonged usage.

Breast cancer is the most common cancer among women in the United States. The lifetime risk of a woman developing breast cancer is 1 in 8. Breast cancer is more common in women older than 50, but it can and does occur in women of all ages. Breast cancer also affects women of all ethnic groups.

The exact cause or causes of breast cancer are still unknown. All women are at risk for developing the disease. Certain factors, however, are known to increase a woman's risk of breast cancer, and other factors are suspected of doing so.

Many of the risk factors that have received coverage in the lay press are associated only with a modest increased risk of breast cancer. A postmenopausal woman age 65, for example, has a relative risk of 5.8 of developing breast cancer simply because of age. This is far greater than the relative risk of developing breast cancer associated with using hormone replacement therapy, which is 1.3 or late menopause, which is 1.2 to 1.5. The highest risks are associated with the presence of germline mutations for breast cancer specific genes or a previous history of biopsy proven atypia, especially if there is a positive family history of breast cancer.

KNOWN RISK FACTORS

Previous Breast Cancer: Women with a history of breast cancer have an increased risk of developing another breast cancer. The risk is about 0.5% to 0.7% per year after diagnosis of the first breast cancer. This means that 10% to 15% of women diagnosed with breast cancer will develop a new cancer in the remaining breast tissue within 20 years.

Family History: Women who have a mother, sister, or daughter with breast cancer have a risk of breast cancer 2 to 4 times greater than average. This risk increases if breast cancer affected a relative at an early age (before menopause), involved both breasts, or was found in several family generations.

BRCA 1 and BRCA 2 Genes: Tumor suppressor genes called BRCA 1 and BRCA 2 are genes that tend to regulate the growth of cells. Women who inherit an abnormal copy of either of these genes have an increased risk of developing breast cancer. BRCA 1 is associated with a higher proportion of inherited breast and ovarian cancers. BRCA 2 is associated with a higher percentage of male breast cancers. Having the abnormal gene does not ensure the certainty of developing breast cancer. Careful follow-up with a genetic counselor or breast specialist is recommended to determine the appropriate treatment options.

Reproductive History: Women who have never been pregnant or who have never given birth to a child and women who have their first child after the age of 30 are usually considered to have 2 to 4 times the average risk of breast cancer.

Women who start having menstrual periods before age 12 and women who have late menopause have about $1\frac{1}{2}$ times the average risk of breast cancer.

Benign Breast Disease: Most benign breast diseases, including *cysts* and benign tumors called *fibroadenomas,* do not increase the risk of breast cancer. However, women with certain benign breast diseases have an increased risk of breast cancer. In particular, women with moderate or severe *hyperplasia,* a condition in which there is an abnormal increase in the number of cells in the breast, have 1.5 to 4 times the average risk of breast cancer. If the extra cells look abnormal, the risk ranges from 3 to 5 times the average and goes as high as 11 times the average if the woman has a family history of breast cancer in first-degree relatives.

CONTROVERSIAL RISK FACTORS

Diet: Some studies have found that diets high in fat or low in fiber increase the risk of breast cancer. These results, however, need to be tested in further studies. In the meantime, women should try to follow the National Cancer Institute's recommendations for a well-balanced diet with three servings per day of fruits and vegetables.

Hormones: Studies have shown a slightly increased risk of breast cancer for women who take hormone replacement therapy (HRT) for long periods of time.

Myth

Breast cancer does not occur in young women.

Fact

Breast cancer is more common in women older than 50, but it can and does occur in women of all ages.

Myth

Women with large breasts have a greater risk of having breast cancer.

Fact

Size has no relation to risk. It is, however, sometimes more difficult to examine large breasts because there is more tissue to mask a lump.

Myth

An injury to the breast can cause breast cancer.

Fact

Cancer is not caused by hurting or bruising the breast. However, when a cancer is already present, it is often detected when a woman touches her breast after an injury.

Myth

Breast-feeding prevents breast cancer.

Fact

Breast-feeding has many benefits, but it reduces the risk of breast cancer very little, if at all.

The benefits of HRT in postmenopausal women—it lowers the risk of fractures due to osteoporosis (brittle bones) and controls hot flashes—should be carefully weighed against the increased risk of breast cancer. For women whose menopausal symptoms are mild to moderate, alternative treatment approaches may be preferable. Every woman considering HRT should discuss her health risks with her primary care physician or gynecologist.

FACTORS THAT DO NOT INCREASE RISK

Injury to the breast is not known to cause breast cancer but often brings the woman's attention to the presence of a pre-existing lump or change. Pregnancy, a condition with very high levels of estrogen, has not been shown to increase the risk of recurrence or new breast cancers in women with a previous history of breast cancer. Breast-feeding reduces the risk of breast cancer very little, if at all.

Remember, risk factors only increase the risk that a cancer may develop at some point in a woman's life. Even so, the majority of women with breast cancer have none of the previously mentioned risk factors.

REDUCING BREAST CANCER RISK

Women who have a high risk of developing breast cancer may want to consider taking an *antiestrogen drug* to help prevent the formation of new tumors. This treatment is called *chemoprevention*. A national study of more than 13,000 high-risk women found that taking the antiestrogen drug tamoxifen (Nolvadex) for 5 years reduced the occurrence of new invasive breast cancers by almost 50%. There are some possible side effects from taking tamoxifen for a long period of time, including an increased risk of endometrial cancer, blood clots in the leg or lung, and possibly stroke. A chemoprevention trial is under way with an antiestrogen drug called raloxifene (Evista). Raloxifene has already been approved by the FDA for the prevention of osteoporosis in postmenopausal women. This chemoprevention study, called the STAR trial (for "Study of Tamoxifen and Raloxifene"), will see if raloxifene is as effective as tamoxifen in preventing new breast cancers, but with fewer side effects. ❧

How Is Breast Cancer Detected?

Detecting breast cancer early, before it has grown very large or spread to other sites, is important. The earlier a breast cancer is detected, the better the chance it can be cured. There are three main methods of detecting breast cancer: *mammography,* breast examination by a doctor or nurse, and *breast self-examination.* Ultrasound (sonography) may be helpful when used in combination with mammography to determine if an abnormality is cystic (benign) or solid (sometimes cancerous).

Myth

Cancer cannot be found unless a lump is felt.

Fact

Mammography can detect early cancers before a lump can be felt.

MAMMOGRAPHY

Mammography is the use of *X-rays* to make pictures of a breast. An X-ray of a breast is called a mammogram. Mammography can detect cancers that are too small to be felt.

For women who have no symptoms of disease, the standard mammography examination includes two X-rays of each breast, one from above and one from the side. To get the best X-ray image, the breast is flattened between two plastic plates (Figure 3).

This compression may be uncomfortable, but it is not harmful to the breast and is usually not painful. Scheduling the mammogram after the menstrual period, when the breasts are less tender, will reduce the discomfort.

The mammograms are read by a *radiologist,* a doctor who specializes in interpreting X-rays. Sometimes the radiologist will use a computer to study a mammographic image. The radiologist looks for signs of possible cancer: areas of tissue distortion or masses, differences between the breasts,

FIGURE 3

Mammography

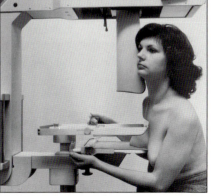

Myth

Mammography is painful and can harm the breast.

Fact

During mammography, the breast is compressed. Although this can be uncomfortable, it is not harmful to the breast and is usually not painful. Scheduling the mammogram after the menstrual period, when the breasts are less tender, will reduce the discomfort.

and abnormal calcium deposits. On a mammogram, a breast cancer often appears as an irregular mass with finger-like extensions. A very early breast cancer sometimes appears as clusters of tiny calcium deposits, called *calcifications*, that are found in an area of rapidly dividing cells. (The appearance of calcium deposits on a mammogram is not related to the amount of calcium in one's diet.) Talcum powder, body cream, and deodorants can contain silica particles that look like calcifications. Therefore, women should not apply these products to the breast or armpit area the day of the mammogram.

A change from one mammogram to the next is sometimes a sign of breast cancer. If a woman had her previous mammograms done at a different facility, she should bring them with her when she has the new mammogram so they will be available to the radiologist for comparison. It is important to choose a mammography facility that meets certain quality standards. The facility should have radiologists and technologists who are specially trained in performing and interpreting mammograms. It should also have a mammography machine that produces high-quality X-rays with a small amount of radiation. One way to determine if a facility meets these standards is to find out whether it is accredited by the American College of Radiology.

Women 40 years or older should have a mammogram every year. Studies show that if all women in this age group had yearly mammograms, the number of women 40 and older who died of breast cancer would be reduced by 25% to 30%.

Although most mammography today preserves breast images on photographic film, a new type of machine uses *digital mammography* in which images are saved as electronic computer files. Digital mammograms are not better than conventional film mammograms for detecting breast cancer, but they do have several advantages. Because the image is an electronic file, it can easily and quickly be sent to a another location. A mammogram ordered by a general practitioner in a small town, for instance, could be sent to breast cancer experts for evaluation. If a radiologist finds a suspicious area on a digital mammogram, that area can be enlarged and electronically enhanced.

BREAST EXAMINATION BY A DOCTOR OR NURSE

All women should have regular breast examinations by a doctor or nurse. In a breast exam, the doctor or nurse looks carefully at the woman's breasts while she sits with her arms relaxed at her sides, then raised over her head, and then flexed, pushing against her hips. The examiner looks for changes in nipple direction and in the symmetry, size, color, and contour of the breasts. The examiner also looks for dimpling or puckering of the skin, scaling of the nipple, and discharge from the nipple. These changes do not always indicate cancer but should always be evaluated. After looking at the breasts, the doctor or nurse palpates (feels) the breasts, chest, supraclavicular (collarbone) area, and axilla (armpit) on each side. Palpation is done while the woman is sitting and again while she is lying down. A skilled examiner can detect subtle changes in the breasts that the woman herself might not notice.

BREAST SELF-EXAMINATION

Beginning around age 20, all women are encouraged to examine their breasts once a month to check for unusual lumps or other signs of cancer. Most women have some lumps in their breasts, especially in the upper outer areas. It is important for women to become familiar with the usual feel and appearance of their breasts so they can detect changes.

Changes are sometimes subtle, and the woman herself may be the first person to detect them. Any change in the breast should be evaluated by a doctor or nurse to make sure it is not breast cancer. Complete instructions for performing breast self-examination are given in the Appendix.

Myth

A breast cancer will always be painless.

Fact

Most early breast cancers do not hurt. However, some are associated with unusual sensations in the breast including soreness or burning.

RECOMMENDATIONS FOR SCREENING EXAMINATIONS

Test	Age	Frequency
Breast self-examination	Begin by age 20	Monthly
Breast examination by a doctor or nurse	20 and older	Annually as part of a complete physical exam
Mammography	Younger than 40	Depending on physical findings, family history, and doctor's recommendation
	40 and older	Annually

*I discovered
my breast cancer
when I was
taking a bath.
I ran my
hand across
my breast and
realized I had a
thickness there.*

Early detection of breast cancer requires cooperation between the woman and her doctor. In addition to maintaining a healthy lifestyle including exercise and a low-fat diet, all women should perform regular breast self-examinations, have regularly scheduled mammograms, and have an annual physical exam that includes a breast exam by a doctor or nurse. A suggested plan is provided in the table on the preceding page.

How Is Breast Cancer Diagnosed?

Most lumps and abnormalities in the breast are caused not by cancer but by benign breast conditions, including *cysts, fibrocystic breast disease, fibroadenomas, fat necrosis,* and *papillomas.* Figures 4–8 illustrate the differences between several benign breast diseases and early breast cancer. When a lump or abnormality is detected, it is important to determine whether it is caused by breast cancer or a benign breast disease.

BENIGN BREAST DISEASES

Cysts are fluid-filled sacs in the breast that generally become larger and painful a week or so before the menstrual period begins. Cysts are quite common in women before menopause. Sometimes a doctor will remove the fluid from a cyst using a syringe with a small needle. For some women, the discomfort of breast cysts can be relieved by reducing the amount of caffeine in the diet. Low-dose vitamin E sometimes gives relief as well. Women with recurrent cysts need to be examined carefully on a regular basis to distinguish new cysts from possible cancers.

Fibrocystic breast disease is another common benign breast condition. In this disease, there is an overgrowth of fibrous tissue in the breast. This extra tissue can feel like lumps, which may appear at any time during the menstrual cycle. Sometimes there are cysts in addition to the overgrowth of fibrous tissue.

The most common solid benign conditions are fibroadenoma and fat necrosis. Fibroadenomas are benign tumors composed of fibrous tissue. On physical examination, they feel smooth, movable, and rubbery. Fat necrosis occurs when fat degenerates, resulting in the development of hard, solid lumps in the breast. Fat necrosis is often the result of a blow to the breast. Fibroadenomas and fat necrosis are more

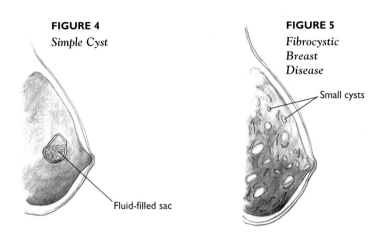

FIGURE 4
Simple Cyst

Fluid-filled sac

FIGURE 5
Fibrocystic Breast Disease

Small cysts

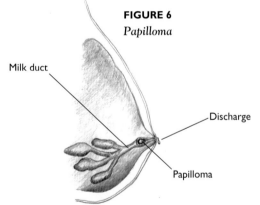

FIGURE 6
Papilloma

Milk duct

Discharge

Papilloma

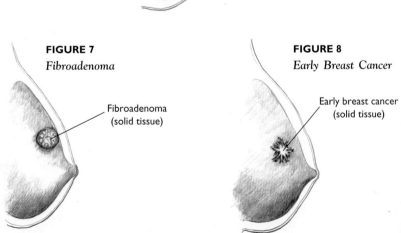

FIGURE 7
Fibroadenoma

Fibroadenoma
(solid tissue)

FIGURE 8
Early Breast Cancer

Early breast cancer
(solid tissue)

common in premenopausal than postmenopausal women. When either type of lump is found in a postmenopausal woman, the lump should be closely monitored to rule out cancer.

Occasionally, women will experience nipple discharge. Because the breast is a gland, secretions from the nipple are not always abnormal. Certain medications, including hormones, can cause occasional nipple discharge. However, should a discharge be noticed, particularly if it comes from only one breast, it should be reported to the doctor. A nipple discharge is generally not a symptom of cancer, but it must be evaluated. A sample of the fluid from the nipple can be smeared on a slide and sent to a laboratory for diagnosis (Figure 9). A benign condition called papilloma, a tiny wart-like growth in a duct of the breast, is the usual cause of an amber or bloody nipple discharge in young women.

Several exams are useful in determining whether a lump or abnormality is benign or malignant.

A new diagnostic test also examines fluid taken from the breast. In this case, the patient massages her breast, squeezing down toward the tip of the nipple. A salt solution is then used to wash cells out of the ducts in the nipple. This test may be able to detect very early breast cancer, or even premalignant cells before they become cancerous. Women in whom premalignant cells are detected may be good candidates for *chemoprevention.*

If the mammography report comes back as "negative," there is nothing else to worry about.

Mammograms do not show 10% to 15% of all breast cancers. Any suspicious mass must be further investigated.

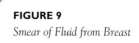

FIGURE 9
Smear of Fluid from Breast

A breast lump must be surgically removed to find out if it is malignant.

Many breast cancers can be diagnosed without a surgical procedure.

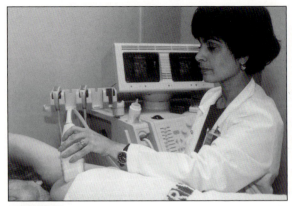

FIGURE 10
Ultrasonography

ULTRASONOGRAPHY

Ultrasonography is used to confirm the presence or absence of a mass and to tell the difference between solid masses and cysts. Ultrasonography (also called ultrasound or sonography) uses high-frequency sound waves to scan the tissue of the breast. Gel is applied to the breast, and a small device called a transducer is slid over the surface of the breast (Figure 10). The transducer produces sound waves, and the way the sound waves travel through the mass indicates whether it is a cyst or solid tumor. The entire process is viewed on a video screen, and photographs are made of significant views.

Unlike mammography, ultrasound uses no radiation. Ultrasound cannot detect very early cancers, so it is best used as an aid in diagnosis rather than as a screening tool for breast cancer.

BIOPSY

If the doctor suspects that a mass is breast cancer, he or she may perform a *biopsy*. In a biopsy, a piece of tissue is removed and examined under a microscope. There are several kinds of biopsy.

Fine-Needle Aspiration and Core Biopsy: In *fine-needle aspiration* (also called FNA) and *core biopsies*, needles are used to remove the tissue. Both procedures are done while the woman is awake, and they do not involve surgical cutting of the breast. If the mass is difficult to feel, ultrasound is sometimes used to guide the needle to ensure that the cells come directly from the tumor.

Before either type of needle biopsy is performed, the breast skin above the lump is cleaned with an antiseptic solution. The patient may be given a local anesthetic to prevent discomfort. In FNA, a fine needle is inserted into the lump, and cells are drawn into the needle (Figure 11). The cells are then pushed out of the needle onto a slide for examination by a *pathologist*. An FNA may be uncomfortable but should not cause any prolonged pain. In a core biopsy, the needle is larger and there is more tissue manipulation. A core biopsy may be done when the physician desires additional tissue to learn more of the characteristics about a tumor such as invasiveness as opposed to noninvasive tumors. If a woman has previously had radiation treatments to her breast, a core biopsy is recommended over a fine-needle aspiration.

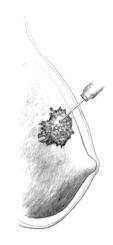

FIGURE 11
Fine-Needle Aspiration

Sometimes fluid is withdrawn with the cells when an FNA is done. If the fluid is straw-colored or dark green (not bloody) and the mass completely disappears when the fluid is withdrawn, then the mass is probably a cyst. In many cases, no further treatment is required. However, if the fluid is bloody or the mass does not completely disappear when the fluid is withdrawn, cancer may be present. When this is the case, the fluid is smeared on a slide and examined under a microscope for cancer cells. This is called a cytological examination.

If a solid mass is detected and an FNA or core biopsy shows no malignant cells, there may still be a tumor. If the doctor, nurse, or patient is concerned about a mass, it must be removed entirely by an excisional biopsy so that all of the mass, not just cells from one portion, can be evaluated.

Why would an FNA or core biopsy miss a tumor? If the tumor is very dense, the needle may not be able to dislodge any malignant cells. A small tumor or an easily movable one can be missed by the needle unless ultrasound guidance is used.

It was important for me to have all the information that I needed about my diagnosis, and then I was able to better make decisions about my treatment.

I had a mammogram in the fall 3 years ago, and they didn't like the way it looked. So they decided that they would do a biopsy. I went in and had the biopsy, and they said they would let me know the next day. My husband and I went the next day, and the doctor came in and put his hand on my shoulder and said, 'I hate to tell you, but you have a malignancy.' We were just devastated—we wished we could have left the room and played like it wasn't us. But I visited with my doctor and also decided I would get a second opinion, which I did. And we went from there.

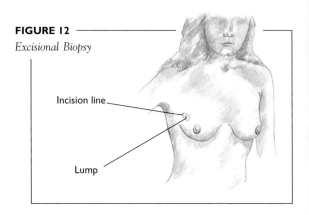

FIGURE 12

Excisional Biopsy

Incision line

Lump

Excisional Biopsy: In an *excisional biopsy* (Figure 12) (also called open biopsy), the entire mass is removed by surgery. This procedure can frequently be done in an outpatient surgical center using only local anesthesia. The entire mass is cut into thin sections and examined by a pathologist over several days. Excisional biopsy is sometimes the most reliable means of diagnosis.

Needle Localization Biopsy: Sometimes, mammography detects calcifications in the breast. These tiny calcium deposits are common and are usually benign. However, an increase in the number of calcifications or clustering of calcifications over time can signal the development of a very early breast cancer. Calcifications are so small they cannot be felt. Sometimes, additional mammograms with the aid of a magnifying glass help the radiologist see them better. If the calcifications are suggestive of breast cancer, a *needle localization biopsy* is done. The radiologist takes an X-ray of the breast and places a thin needle in the center of the group of calcifications. The surgeon then removes the needle and surrounding tissue. Another X-ray is made of the excised tissue to ensure that all of the calcifications have been removed. The final diagnosis is available in about a week after the pathologist has carefully looked at all of the tissue placed on slides under the microscope.

ॐ

How Is Breast Cancer Treated?

When a woman has been diagnosed with breast cancer, she and her team of doctors develop a comprehensive treatment plan. This team may include a *medical oncologist, radiation oncologist*, and/or a *surgical oncologist* as well as other health professionals. The treatment plan outlines the type of surgery that will be used to remove the tumor and any additional therapy, such as *radiation therapy, chemotherapy*, or *hormonal therapy*, that will be given. The plan also specifies whether the woman will have *reconstructive surgery*. There are many different types of breast cancer, so the treatment is not the same for every woman. The treatment depends upon many factors including the type of cancer cells, how much the disease has spread, and the size of the tumor in relation to the breast. The size of the tumor combined with the known or suspected spread of disease to other parts of the body determines the sequencing of treatment. Often cancers of the breast larger than 2 centimeters will be treated with systemic therapy (chemotherapy) before surgery to reduce the size of the cancer and to measure the tumor response to the chemotherapy agent(s) used. If the tumor is not shrinking on one chemotherapy regimen, another may be substituted for more effective results. Remember that chemotherapy is a systemic treatment, meaning it affects cancer cells throughout the body. Thus, the breast tumor cells are being destroyed at the same time as other cancer cells that might have escaped the breast and are seeking other body sites in which to grow.

Myth

Removal of the entire breast is safer than segmental mastectomy and radiation therapy.

Fact

Survival is similar for patients who have breast-conserving therapy and those who undergo total or modified radical mastectomy.

SURGERY

There are three main surgical treatments for breast cancer: *modified radical mastectomy, total mastectomy*, and *segmental (partial) mastectomy*. These may also include sentinel node biopsy with or without axillary node dissection.

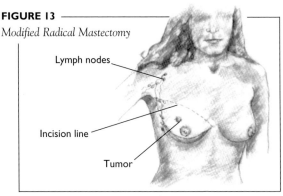

FIGURE 13

Modified Radical Mastectomy

Lymph nodes

Incision line

Tumor

For a person who's facing being told that now she has cancer . . . I think you have this fantasy that it's a dream, and you're going to wake up. And then you realize that it's not a dream, it's reality—and you're faced with having to make decisions quickly because you have to get started on treatment.

Modified Radical Mastectomy: In a standard modified radical mastectomy (Figure 13), the entire breast (including the nipple) and some, but not all, of the lymph nodes from the armpit (the *axillary lymph nodes*) are removed. The chest muscles are not removed, so the chest is smooth and flat after surgery. Surgeons prefer to make a diagonal incision. This ensures that the scar will not be visible in low-cut clothing and allows a *prosthesis* to fit more comfortably. Frequently, immediate reconstruction is done as part of the same surgical procedure. This eliminates the need for a prosthesis.

Total Mastectomy: In a total mastectomy (Figure 14), the entire breast (including the nipple and surrounding areola) are removed, but the axillary lymph nodes are not removed. This type of surgery is typically performed for noninvasive breast cancers (cancers that do not infiltrate and destroy healthy cells or tissues). As with a modified radical mastectomy, surgeons prefer to make a diagonal incision.

FIGURE 14

Total Mastectomy

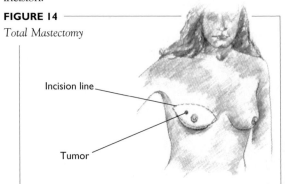

Incision line

Tumor

Segmental Mastectomy: In a segmental mastectomy (also referred to as partial mastectomy or lumpectomy) (Figure 15), the surgeon removes only the tumor and a small amount of surrounding breast tissue. The size of the tumor is the main factor determining the appropriateness of this type of surgery. The shape and location of the incision usually depend upon the woman's anatomy and the location of the tumor in the breast. Sometimes a *sentinel node biopsy* with or without an axillary node dissection is recommended. The nodes are removed through a separate incision in the armpit. The shape of the breast is changed very little after a segmental mastectomy, so a prosthesis or breast reconstruction is not needed. A segmental mastectomy is usually followed by 5 to 6 weeks of radiation therapy. The combination of segmental mastectomy and radiation therapy is often referred to as *breast-conserving therapy*. Chemotherapy may also be recommended by your physician following a segmental mastectomy.

Axillary Lymph Node Dissection: In an *axillary lymph node dissection*, some of the nodes in the armpit are removed. The nodes themselves are embedded in fatty tissue and difficult to see, so the surgeon removes a portion of the fatty tissue, and then a pathologist carefully separates the nodes from the rest of the tissue. The nodes are examined under a microscope to find out if they contain cancer cells. This is the best way to determine *prognosis* and any necessary additional treatment, such as chemotherapy or hormonal therapy.

My sentinel node had a microscopic spot of cancer. Neither the ultrasound nor the physical exams indicated the presence of any cancer in my lymph nodes, so I am very glad that we went ahead and did the sentinel node biopsy.

FIGURE 15

Segmental Mastectomy

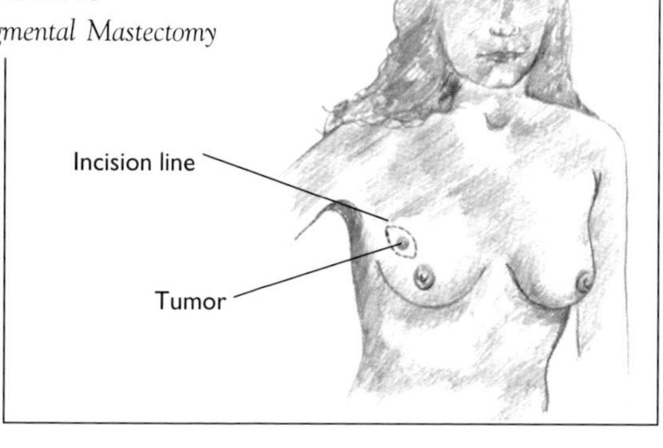

Incision line

Tumor

Myth

It is always necessary to surgically remove the lymph nodes in the armpit in order to determine if they contain cancer cells.

Fact

Sentinel Node Biopsy can tell your doctor if the cancer cells have spread to your axillary nodes, and may make an axillary node dissection unnecessary.

The results of the pathologist's examination are usually available within a week. If the nodes contain cancer cells, *adjuvant therapy* will be recommended. If the nodes do not contain cancer cells, the decision about whether to use adjuvant therapy will depend on a variety of factors, including the size of the cancer, the patient's age, and whether the tumor is sensitive to estrogen.

After an axillary node dissection, fluid can collect in the arm and hand on the treatment side and cause them to become swollen. This condition is called *lymphedema*. However, with less radical surgery and careful attention to the proper use of the hand and arm on the affected side, lymphedema is not common and usually not severe. With the limited axillary dissections that are typically used today, the likelihood of developing lymphedema is less than 10%.

Sentinel Node Biopsy: Sentinel Node Biopsy (SNB) is a new advance in the treatment of breast cancer. It is a relatively simple procedure (Figure 16) which may reduce the amount of surgery needed for staging and treatment of early breast cancer. Part of the SNB procedure is Lymph Node Mapping. This is a means by which your doctor can detect the pattern of lymph drainage from your tumor and identify the node or nodes most likely to contain cancer cells if they have escaped from the breast. The lymph nodes are part of the body's infection-fighting system and are located throughout your body. A fluid called lymph flows through these nodes. The nodes act as a filter to decrease spread of bacteria. This same lymph system is the route for cancer cells to leave the breast and spread to other body parts. When malignant (cancer) cells

FIGURE 16

Sentinel Node Biopsy

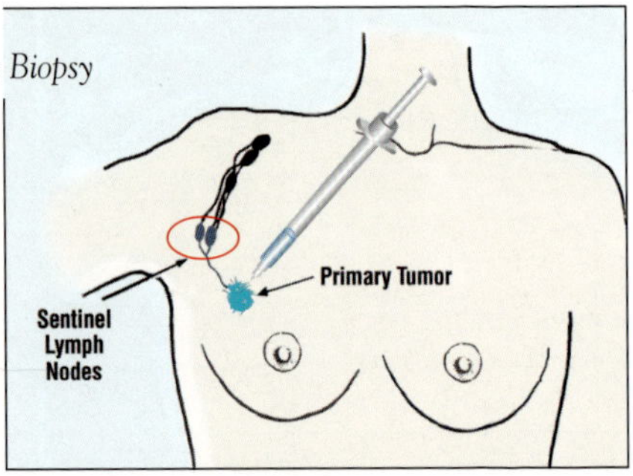

Primary Tumor

Sentinel Lymph Nodes

reach the lymph system, they multiply. From there they can pass into the bloodstream. In the case of a breast cancer, the lymph flow is usually to the nodes in the axilla or armpit. The sentinel nodes are the first nodes through which lymphatic fluid flows from a breast tumor. These nodes are the gatekeepers for the remainder of the axillary nodes.

Intraoperative Lymph Node Mapping with Sentinel Node Biopsy (IOLM-SNB), commonly called Sentinel Node Biopsy, can tell your doctor if the cancer cells have spread to your axillary nodes. If the sentinel node(s) are negative for cancer cells, an axillary node dissection may not be necessary. When the node(s) have cancer cells in them, it will be important to remove more nodes to determine the extent of spread and plan for additional systemic treatment.

Recovering From Surgery: Many women are able to leave the hospital the day after surgery. Some women, however, must remain in the hospital for a few days. After the first 24 hours, pain and discomfort can usually be relieved with oral pain medication.

During surgery, *drains* are placed in the wound site to collect fluid. The drains used for breast surgery are usually made of tubing and suction bottles. One end of the tubing is placed under the skin in the wound site; the other is left outside the body and connected to a suction bottle. Drains are usually left in place for about 10 days after surgery. The site where the tubing enters the skin must be cleaned each day, and the collection bottles must be emptied twice a day. The patient and her caregivers are taught drain care before surgery. When there is minimal drainage for 2 consecutive days, the patient returns to the hospital, and the drains are removed. This procedure is performed without anesthesia. The patient may feel some stinging when the drains are removed but will not feel prolonged pain.

Most women who have a modified radical mastectomy or a segmental mastectomy with an axillary lymph node dissection are able to return to their normal activities within 3 to 4 weeks. As soon as the drains are removed, range of motion exercises should begin to ensure the return to full activities.

*M*yth

Once the lymph nodes are removed from the armpit, there will always be swelling of the arm.

*F*act

Some women experience swelling of the affected arm (lymphedema). However, with less radical surgery and careful attention to the proper use of the hand and arm on the affected side, swelling is not common and usually not severe.

I would recommend this procedure called Sentinel Node Biopsy to a friend who had the same situation. In my experience, after surgery I had no complications, infections, or swelling of the arm, and my recovery time was short.

Myth

Women with a strong family history of breast cancer should not consider breast-conserving therapy.

Fact

A strong family history of breast cancer is not a contraindication to breast-conserving therapy. The decision about which treatment to use should take into account several factors such as stage of the breast cancer, body build, and lifestyle.

GUIDELINES FOR BREAST-CONSERVING THERAPY

Women who are offered breast-conserving therapy may wonder if it is better to have a mastectomy instead to prevent a recurrence of cancer. Several studies have shown that women who have breast-conserving therapy live as long and remain free of cancer as those who have a mastectomy.

In general, women who desire to preserve their breast, are willing to come for daily outpatient radiation treatments over 5 to 6 weeks, and are able to return for regular check-ups can have breast-conserving therapy. However, mastectomy may be more appropriate for certain women. The woman and her doctors should consider several factors when choosing between breast-conserving therapy and mastectomy.

The size of the tumor, the presence of disease elsewhere in the body, and a woman's personal preference should all be taken into consideration when weighing surgical options. For breast-conserving therapy, the breast must be large enough that the tumor and some healthy tissue around it can be removed with a reasonable cosmetic result. No woman is too young or old to have breast-conserving therapy. Women with lupus erythematosus or scleroderma may not be able to tolerate irradiation of the skin and therefore may not be able to have breast-conserving therapy.

A strong family history of breast cancer does not mean that a woman cannot undergo breast-conserving therapy. The woman should be counseled regarding her individual risk for a second breast cancer in either breast, especially if the family history involves several close family members with breast cancer, or any relative with breast cancer before menopause or with bilateral breast cancers.

RECONSTRUCTIVE SURGERY

For women who need or prefer to have a modified radical or total mastectomy, surgery to reconstruct a breast mound is a treatment option. The reconstruction can be performed either at the time of mastectomy (*immediate reconstruction*) or later (*delayed reconstruction*).

Immediate reconstruction has several advantages. First, there is less psychological trauma because the woman does not have to live without a breast mound for any length of time. Second, only one operation is necessary. This is important because general anesthesia always carries a very small risk of serious complications. Third, the cosmetic result of immediate reconstruction is often better because some of the breast skin can be preserved and incorporated into the new breast mound.

Immediate reconstruction, however, is not appropriate for all patients. Breast reconstruction should be delayed if the patient is unsure about having the operation, if complex postoperative radiation therapy is being considered, or if prolonged anesthesia will unduly increase the operative risk.

Breast reconstruction can be performed using either *implants* or the patient's own tissue. Implants are silicone bags filled with salt water or silicone gel that are surgically placed beneath the skin or muscle of the chest. The main advantage of implants is that they can be inserted quickly and easily, so operating time is relatively short. However, implants have several disadvantages: they can cause an infection; they can rupture; and the salt water or silicone gel can leak out. Implants can also cause capsular contracture, a hardening of the tissue around the implant. Another disadvantage is that for most women, the chest tissue must be stretched over a period of 4 to 6 months before the implant can be inserted. In addition, how long implants will last before they need to be replaced is not yet known.

For these reasons, the use of the patient's own tissue has become the method of choice for breast reconstruction. In this type of reconstruction, a flap of muscle and skin (a *myocutaneous flap*) is taken from another part of the body and used to reconstruct a breast mound. There are several kinds of flaps, each one named for the muscle it comes from. The two main flaps used in breast reconstruction are the latissimus dorsi flap (Figure 17), taken from the back just below the shoulder, and the transverse rectus abdominis myocutaneous (TRAM) flap (Figure 18), which is taken from the

Before I even started my treatment, I was fortunate enough to meet a woman who had reconstruction and see the work that had been done on her. I was just fascinated that it could look so remarkably normal. So for me it was an easy decision to go with reconstruction. I wanted my breasts back, however I could get them. This was an option, and I said, 'Great!'

yth

Women should not have immediate breast reconstruction. It is best to wait a couple of years to make sure the cancer does not recur.

act

With proper surgical removal of the cancer in the breast, there is no reason to delay reconstruction in most patients. In fact, immediate reconstruction is often preferable since only one surgery is required and the cosmetic results can be better.

FIGURE 17

Latissimus Dorsi Flap Reconstruction

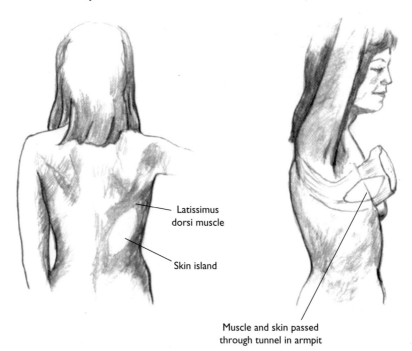

Latissimus
dorsi muscle

Skin island

Muscle and skin passed
through tunnel in armpit

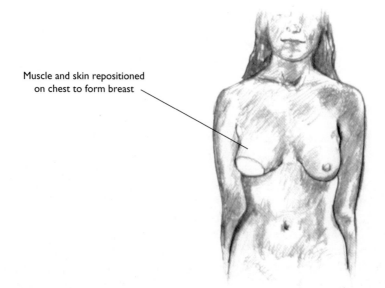

Muscle and skin repositioned
on chest to form breast

abdomen. The TRAM flap is sometimes called the "tummy tuck" flap because the fatty tissue from the stomach is used to create a breast mound. In some cases, a flap is rotated to cover the mastectomy site without cutting the blood vessels. In other cases, the vessels are cut and reconnected using microscopic instruments.

Women having immediate breast reconstruction may be eligible for a skin-sparing mastectomy which allows for removal of less breast skin. This generally includes removal of the nipple-areola complex and skin overlying the tumor or biopsy site. An effort is made to save as much of the breast skin as possible which becomes an envelope for the reconstructive tissue.

If the woman desires nipple reconstruction, it is usually performed later using nearby skin flaps. The reconstructed nipple and the skin around it (the areola) are tattooed with a color that matches the opposite nipple and areola.

The sensations in a reconstructed breast are not the same as those in a woman's own breast tissue. The sensitivity to touch is diminished. In fact, many women describe a sensation of numbness in the reconstructed breast. However, the reconstructed breast has a normal size, shape, and contour. After TRAM flap reconstruction, the stomach is firm and flat but may be less sensitive to touch. Women who have immediate reconstruction with the TRAM flap generally remain in the hospital about 1 week after surgery and are able to return to work in about 6 to 8 weeks.

Because part of the muscle is actually removed in a TRAM flap, some patients may have abdominal weakness as a long-term side effect. To avoid this problem, a variation of the TRAM flap called the DIEP flap (for Deep Inferior Epigastric Perforator) has recently been developed. The DIEP flap uses skin and fat from the stomach, but does not remove any of the muscle. Although this surgery is more difficult to perform than a regular TRAM flap, recovery time is faster, and the patient can usually go home from

Prior to surgery, I did not see any pictures of what a mastectomy scar looked like. I'm the kind of person that really doesn't want to know what's going to happen to me until after it's done. After surgery, I was amazed when they removed the bandages. You basically have a simple scar, a simple line going across where you once had a breast.

FIGURE 18

TRAM Flap Reconstruction

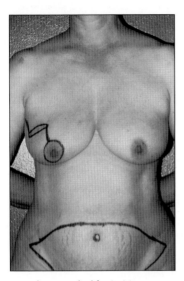

Areas marked for incision
prior to procedure

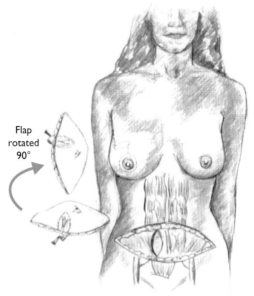

Flap
rotated
90°

Abdominal tissue used to create breast mound;
nearby skin flap used to reconstruct nipple

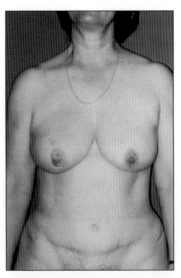

After recovery from procedure, a new
reconstructed nipple and areola are
tattooed to match opposite breast

the hospital much sooner. Because DIEP flap reconstruction is relatively new, it is not yet available at all institutions.

RADIATION THERAPY

In radiation therapy (Figure 19), high-energy rays are used to destroy cancer cells by injuring their ability to multiply. Radiation therapy is usually given after segmental mastectomy to sterilize any cancer cells that might be left in the breast. It does not make the patient radioactive.

Treatments are generally given during daily clinic visits over 5 to 6 weeks. Each radiation treatment takes only about 2 to 5 minutes. Before the first treatment, the patient undergoes a simulated radiation treatment. She lies on a table under the machine that will deliver the radiation, and a technician marks the areas that will be irradiated (Figure 20). The markings are made with indelible ink, and they are left on during the entire 5 to 6 weeks of treatment to ensure that the same area is irradiated every time. During this time, the patient must take sponge baths instead of showers to make sure the markings are not erased. (Sometimes small tattoos are used instead of ink markings.)

Radiation treatment is not painful. Some women experience tingling or warmth in the treated area. Others report feeling more tired than usual and decrease their activity during the weeks of daily treatments. For fair-skinned women whose skin burns easily from the sun, wearing a clean cotton T-shirt is usually more comfortable than wearing a bra during the weeks of treatment.

The treated breast is usually somewhat firmer and slightly smaller after treatment than before. The skin may become thicker. In some women, the breast becomes larger because of fluid buildup within the breast tissue. Radiation therapy usually causes a subtle darkening of the skin in the treated area. Some women apply aloe vera cream to the treated area to keep it soft.

The radiation started about a month after my surgery. First I had to go in for the markings to pinpoint where they were going to do the radiation. That took 3 or 4 hours. Then every day I would go in the afternoon. I would change into a gown and be brought into the radiation room, where I would lie down in a certain position. The radiation took about half a minute. Then I would have to change into another position and they would change the machine into another position. After another half a minute of radiation, I was finished and I could get dressed and go.

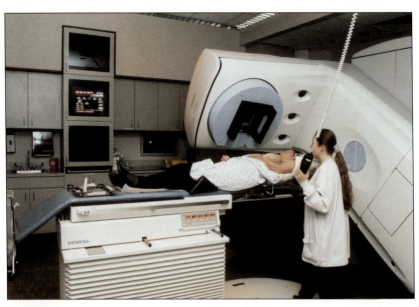

FIGURE 19
Radiation Therapy to the Breast

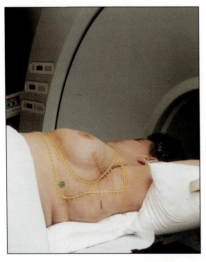

FIGURE 20
Marking Breast Area for Irradiation

Radiation therapy is usually not needed after a modified radical or total mastectomy except for women who have advanced cancers and are at high risk for having the breast cancer recur on the chest wall.

CHEMOTHERAPY

Chemotherapy is the use of drugs to damage or kill cancer cells. Chemotherapy for breast cancer patients usually lasts 3 to 6 months. Depending on the type of chemotherapy, the patient receives drugs during part of each month, followed by a rest period. This rest period gives the body a chance to recover from the effects of the chemotherapy.

Chemotherapy drugs can be given by mouth, by injection, or by infusion into a vein. Often the drugs are given through a flexible tube called a *central venous catheter*. The tube is inserted into a large vein (usually under the patient's collarbone) before treat-

FIGURE 21

Chemotherapy Through a Central Venous Catheter

Subclavian vein into which catheter is inserted

Exit site through skin (exposed catheter)

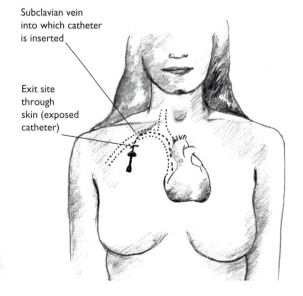

Radiation therapy burns and destroys the skin of the breast.

Fact

The X-rays used to treat breast cancer can cause temporary redness of the skin much like a sunburn. This can be soothed with an ointment and diminishes after the completion of treatment.

Myth

Women receiving radiation therapy should avoid physical contact with friends and family because of possible radioactivity.

The form of X-ray energy used to treat breast cancer does not linger in the body. Other than slight tenderness of the treated areas, there is no reason to avoid physical contact with others.

Myth

Once a woman has been treated for breast cancer, she should avoid becoming pregnant.

Fact

Pregnancy need not be avoided by women who are free of cancer and not undergoing treatment. Successful pregnancies have occurred even in women who have undergone abdominal surgery for a TRAM-flap reconstruction.

ment begins (Figure 21). The tube is left in place during the entire period of chemotherapy. When drugs are not being given, the tube is sealed and taped to the chest.

Chemotherapy can be given in a hospital, a clinic, or a doctor's office. Most patients are able to go home between treatments and during the recovery period, but some women need to stay in the hospital during treatment. Chemotherapy can also be given through a portable pump that the patient carries around with her while she goes about her normal activities. The patient comes to the hospital on the first day of treatment, and a small pump is attached to the central venous catheter. The pump dispenses drugs at a steady rate. The patient returns to the hospital at the end of the treatment period (usually about 3 days later), and the pump is removed.

Because chemotherapy affects any cell that is in the process of multiplying, normal cells may also be damaged (but to a lesser degree). Chemotherapy involves the person's entire body and produces a number of side effects. One of the most feared side effects is nausea and vomiting. Fortunately, very effective medications have been developed to reduce the severity of these effects and even prevent them altogether in some patients. Other common side effects are hair loss, increased chance of infections, bleeding of the gums, mouth sores, anemia, and fatigue. In women who have not gone through menopause, chemotherapy often causes changes in the menstrual cycle; sometimes there are no periods at all during therapy. However, it is important to continue to use adequate birth control even if periods have stopped. Hormones in birth control pills can interfere with chemotherapy, so sexually active women must use another form of birth control until all chemotherapy is completed. Most side effects are temporary and go away after the chemotherapy is finished.

Most women are able to continue their normal activities while they are receiving chemotherapy. Some women feel more tired than usual and work half days or part-time.

Chemotherapy is sometimes given as the only treatment if the breast cancer has spread to other parts of the body. More commonly, chemotherapy is given with surgery, radiation therapy, or both to decrease the chance that the cancer will recur. This is done when there is a high risk that tumor cells have spread into the blood or lymph vessels. Chemotherapy given for this purpose is called *adjuvant therapy*. In some cases, chemotherapy may be given before surgery to attempt to reduce the size of the lump and therefore make breast-conserving therapy possible. This type of chemotherapy is sometimes called *neoadjuvant therapy*.

DRUGS COMMONLY USED TO TREAT BREAST CANCER

Oncologists commonly use more than one drug, or what is called combination therapy, to treat breast cancer. They do this because cancer cells can become resistant to individual drugs.

For more than 20 years, oncologists have used a regimen known as CMF (cyclophosphamide, methotrexate, and 5-fluorouracil) in hopes of preventing the recurrence of breast cancer. Studies of patients with positive nodes who received CMF after surgery found they had better outcomes than those who had no chemotherapy. Later studies found that CMF also helped patients with negative nodes when used in the adjuvant setting.

The class of drugs known as anthracyclines (e.g., Adriamycin) has become standard in the treatment of breast cancer. Often, oncologists give the combination of Adriamycin and cyclophosphamide (AC) to patients with positive nodes following surgery. Another popular combination is CAF (cyclophosphamide, Adriamycin, 5-fluorouracil). The same combination of drugs is sometimes used in a different order in a regimen known as FAC. A newer anthracycline, epirubicin (Ellence), is as effective as doxorubicin, but may have fewer side effects. It is also used in combination with cyclophosphamide and 5-fluorouracil (CEF).

Myth

Chemotherapy is given only to women with advanced breast cancer.

Fact

Chemotherapy is now recommended for most women with breast cancer. Even in women with very early disease, it usually improves survival and reduces the possibility of recurrence. Chemotherapy is also given to some women with breast cancer to reduce the size of the tumor before surgery.

You know, you hear all these stories that you're going to lose your hair, so I had it cut relatively short. I sort of lost it in clumps—it doesn't fall out all at once, it's a gradual thing you notice over a period of days. I got tired of seeing it disappear, so I had my head shaved. I did buy several wigs. I just felt it would look more like me if I was wearing a wig instead of a scarf or hat, but when I was at home, I took the wig off. I lost my eyelashes, my eyebrows, every stitch of hair— but it came back.

Patients who take anthracycline-containing regimens experience more of certain side effects, such as hair loss and nausea, but these regimens tend to be more effective at killing cancer cells than CMF.

A newer class of chemotherapy agents is the taxanes, including Taxotere (docetaxel) and paclitaxel, with Taxotere being the more recent advance for the treatment of breast cancer. Most chemotherapy drugs stop cancer cells from dividing by interfering with the cell's DNA, but the taxanes act quite differently. They damage the supporting structure of the tumor cell, which is almost like a skeleton, and in this way prevent the cell from dividing. Recent studies have shown Taxotere to be a very active drug in advanced breast cancer and many patients who do not respond to CMF or a combination of drugs containing Adriamycin respond to Taxotere.

Taxotere is also very effective when it is used in combination with other chemotherapy drugs. Taxotere administered at the same time as Adriamycin and cyclophosphamide (TAC) may have higher response rates than standard FAC chemotherapy. Taxotere administered simultaneously with capecitabine (Xeloda) (a drug that is converted into 5-fluorouracil in the body after taking it orally) results in better outcomes than Taxotere alone.

IMMUNOLOGICAL THERAPY

An exciting new approach for the treatment of breast cancer is the use of antibodies that target specific proteins in cancer cells. A gene called HER-2/neu makes a protein that regulates cell growth by allowing growth factors to enter the cell. About 25% of women with breast cancer have extra HER-2/neu genes in their tumors, and extra copies of the protein on the surface of the tumor cells. Herceptin (trastuzumab) is an antibody that binds to these proteins in a very specific way, like a key going into a lock, and prevents them from allowing the entry of growth factors into the cell. Herceptin treatment has been used chiefly for the treatment of patients with metastatic breast cancer who have not responded well to other treatments. Researchers are also using it in combination with other chemotherapy drugs to see if it will result in a better patient outcome. It is important to remember that Herceptin is only likely to be effective in the 25% of women with extra HER-2/neu genes and protein in their tumor cells.

There are many other proteins in cancer cells that may be good targets for immunological therapy. Someday, it may be possible to treat breast cancer using antibodies that affect only the cancer cells and have none of the unpleasant side effects of chemotherapy.

HORMONAL THERAPY

In hormonal therapy, antiestrogen drugs are used to block the effects of hormones that promote tumor growth. Estrogen is a hormone that sometimes promotes the growth of breast cancer. Antiestrogen drugs are pills taken by mouth daily for a few years following surgery. Hormonal therapy affects the entire body. It can cause hot flashes, excessive perspiration, vaginal itching or bleeding, temporary weight gain, nausea, and occasional depression.

Not all breast cancers are sensitive to estrogen. To determine if a tumor is sensitive to estrogen, an *estrogen receptor assay* (also called an estrogen receptor test or ER test) is performed on cancer tissue removed at the time of surgery. A tumor sensitive to estrogen is estrogen receptor–positive; a tumor that is not sensitive is estrogen receptor–negative. Estrogen-receptor–positive cancers are generally more likely to respond to hormonal therapy; hormonal therapy is usually not used for estrogen-receptor–negative cancers.

AROMATASE INHIBITORS

Another therapy now available for postmenopausal women with estrogen-sensitive breast cancer uses drugs called aromatase inhibitors to lower the amount of estrogen produced by the body. After menopause, estrogen is no longer produced by the ovaries. Instead, it is produced in muscle, skin, fat, and breast cells,

Women who have had breast cancer can never take hormones.

Although this issue is controversial, some women are now given estrogen following treatment of breast cancer if the cancer was early-stage and not sensitive to estrogen.

where another hormone called androgen is converted into estrogen by the enzyme aromatase. Aromatase inhibitors stop the synthesis of estrogen from androgen in postmenopausal women. Several aromatase inhibitors are now being used, including anastrozole (Arimidex), letrozole (Femara), and exemestane (Aromasin). They appear to work at least as well as tamoxifen in preventing the recurrence of breast cancer, with a lower risk of toxic effects that may sometimes be associated with tamoxifen use, such as endometrial cancer, blood clots, and vaginal bleeding. The use of aromatase inhibitors may result in an increased risk of bone fractures and of bone and muscle aches, but these effects are usually modest. Recent studies with exemestane indicate that aromatase inhibitors may provide additional protection against breast cancer recurrence, even in women who have already completed the recommended 5 years of tamoxifen treatment.

Follow-Up Care After Breast Cancer

Good follow-up care (care given after the initial treatment is completed) is essential for all women who have had breast cancer. Good follow-up care includes physical examinations to check for signs of possible recurrence and social and psychological support to help women cope with the long-term effects of diagnosis and treatment.

For most women, one of the greatest difficulties after treatment is the fear of recurrence. Any change in the treated breast or chest wall or elsewhere in the body can cause a woman to become alarmed. It is important to realize, however, that while these changes might be signs of a breast cancer recurrence, they also might be signs of other physical problems. Regular follow-up exams can distinguish between recurrences and other physical problems and ensure that if there is a recurrence, it will be detected early.

GUIDELINES FOR FOLLOW-UP

Follow-up exams can be done by a primary care physician or a nonphysician provider such as a nurse practitioner or physician assistant. It is important to see a doctor or nurse who is sensitive to the fears and concerns of women with a history of breast cancer.

Invasive Breast Cancer: The risk of recurrence for women with invasive breast cancer depends on many factors, including the type of cancer cell and the stage of the cancer at diagnosis. The risk of recurrence is greatest during the first 2 years after treatment and decreases beyond 5 years after the completion of treatment. The longer the time since the completion of treatment, the less likely the cancer is to recur.

In general, women with invasive breast cancer should have a physical exam every 4 months for the

Myth

Any ache or pain noted after treatment of breast cancer should be considered a possible sign of recurrence.

Fact

Your body continues to have common aches and pains, such as those caused by arthritis, regardless of the cancer. It is important to discuss specific *new* sensations with your doctor.

Myth

A woman who has had breast cancer must have bone scans, CT scans, X-rays, and blood tests at least once a year for the rest of her life.

Fact

Although these additional tests may be needed in certain cases, a woman who has remained cancer-free for 5 years usually requires only an annual physical exam and mammogram, and perhaps an annual chest X-ray, if she received radiation therapy as part of her cancer treatment.

first 2 years after treatment and every 6 months for the next 3 years. At these check-ups, the doctor or nurse may request additional tests, depending on whether the patient has any symptoms. Once a woman has remained free of cancer for 5 years after completion of treatment, she requires only an annual physical exam and mammogram and perhaps an annual chest X-ray, if she received radiation therapy. Women who have had breast-conserving therapy need to have annual mammograms of both the treated and untreated breasts. After mastectomy and reconstructive surgery, a mammogram of the reconstructed breast is not necessary.

Noninvasive Breast Cancer: For women with noninvasive breast cancer, the risk of recurrence is very small. Women in this group need only annual physical exams and mammograms, the same care recommended for women who have never had breast cancer.

ESTROGEN

Women with a history of breast cancer should consult with their doctor before taking estrogen in the form of birth control pills or estrogen replacement therapy. There is a great deal of debate about this issue. If the initial tumor was early-stage and not sensitive to estrogen, a woman might be able to take estrogen after the completion of treatment. If the initial tumor was sensitive to estrogen, birth control pills and estrogen replacement therapy are generally not recommended. However, for some women with severe menopausal symptoms, the benefits of estrogen replacement therapy may outweigh the risks. Women should discuss these risks and benefits with a doctor before deciding whether to take estrogen.

২

Coping With Breast Cancer

Breast cancer affects all aspects of a woman's life—not just her physical well-being. The disease affects relationships with family members and friends, feelings about sexuality, and work patterns. Although every person will react differently to the diagnosis of breast cancer and to the effects of treatment, dealing with the emotional impact of breast cancer is essential to the recovery process. Family, friends, doctors, nurses, social workers, and others can all help with emotional as well as physical recovery. The most important thing to remember is that a woman can lead a fulfilling, normal life after having had breast cancer.

FAMILY

Breast cancer affects the entire family. The normal routine is disrupted, and everyone is concerned and experiences emotions such as worry, fear, and anger. For both a woman and her family, talking about the breast cancer can be difficult. The woman may wish to protect her loved ones by hiding the effects of the breast cancer and its treatment and by acting as if life is "normal." Her family members may be afraid to ask questions about the disease.

However, most families find that being open and honest about the disease helps the entire family cope better. Involving the husband or partner and other family members in discussions about diagnosis, treatment options, side effects, and possible outcomes helps the whole family adjust. If the woman wishes, family members can be invited to participate in discussions with doctors.

Women who are used to being caregivers may find it difficult to let others care for them, but it is important to let family members lend their support. If the

yth

It is generally best to make treatment decisions quickly and not to burden other family members in the decision-making process.

act

Breast cancer affects the entire family. Everyone has feelings of concern, fear, and anger because of the disease. It is best to openly discuss all treatment options and possible outcomes. Mutual decision-making can strengthen family relationships and make the post-treatment adjustment much easier for everyone.

There is so much information that you have to absorb, and so many questions that are going through your mind. First of all, are you going to live? And what kind of life are you going to have?

Myth

Women who have breast-conserving therapy rather than modified radical or total mastectomy generally have a more active sex life after treatment.

Fact

Women who have breast-conserving therapy may feel more comfortable with their bodies, particularly when nude. However, there is little difference in marital happiness, frequency of sex, or sexual satisfaction between women who have modified radical or total mastectomies and those who have segmental mastectomies.

woman undergoes surgery, family members can help care for at her at home afterwards. Family members can also help out by taking over any household chores the woman normally does.

CHILDREN

Children are quick to detect changes in the family's routine and to sense tension, anger, and depression. It is important to give children some information about the disease so they will understand the changes occurring around them. It is best to explain the disease in simple terms and to emphasize that the family will try to return to its normal routine as soon as possible. With young children, it is important to emphasize that the child did not cause the mother's illness. Children are naturally curious and may ask to see or touch a mastectomy scar, chemotherapy pump, prosthesis, or some other sign of the breast cancer treatment. Allowing a child to satisfy his or her curiosity may help the child cope better with the breast cancer.

SUPPORT GROUPS

Many women find it helpful to talk with other women who have had breast cancer. Several organizations sponsor support groups (see "Resources for Breast Cancer Patients"). Hospital social workers and family therapists can help identify groups in a woman's community. Friends or relatives who have experienced the disease can also be an excellent source of support.

BODY IMAGE

The physical changes caused by breast cancer treatment may make a woman feel different or isolated from others who have not experienced the disease. For women who have had a mastectomy, a prosthesis can help restore the pretreatment appearance. Mastectomy bras and prostheses (Figure 22) are now sold through catalogues and by several national department store chains. The American Cancer Society's Reach to Recovery volunteers have a selection of prostheses

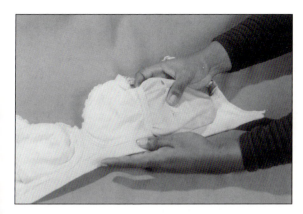

FIGURE 22

Mastectomy Bra and Breast Prosthesis

that women can try on by appointment. Volunteers can also provide a list of prosthesis manufacturers. Some women make their own prosthesis by sewing a fabric backing onto the cup of a regular bra and filling the resulting pocket with a soft material such as pillow stuffing (available at any fabric store).

SEXUALITY

The physical changes brought about by breast cancer treatment can temporarily interfere with a woman's sexuality. Women—especially those who have had a mastectomy—may be uncomfortable undressing in front of a partner or sleeping in the nude. Anxiety about the cancer and its treatment can cause a couple to lose interest in lovemaking. Side effects of treatment can also result in a temporary loss of desire. A woman's partner may be reluctant to engage in sexual activity out of fear of hurting her. Most couples find that by talking about these changes and being patient, their sex life can be just as fulfilling after treatment as it was before.

Several myths still exist that can interfere with a couple's expression of their sexuality. Couples should remember the following facts:

- It is not possible to "catch" cancer from someone else. Cancer is not contagious.

I know you can buy beautiful bras that are custom made for you, but I haven't gone and gotten one yet. It really hasn't bothered me or my husband that I had my right breast removed. Life goes on.

My lifestyle is the same as it was before the cancer was diagnosed. I do anything I want to do. We went tubing down the Guadelupe River for 4$^{1}/_{2}$ hours. I was on that inner tube, paddling along, and it didn't bother me one bit. I do everything I did before.

• It is not possible to "become radioactive" by touching a person who is undergoing radiation therapy. The form of energy used in radiation therapy does not linger in the body. There is no reason for women undergoing radiation therapy to avoid sexual contact.

• Caressing a breast does not lead to cancer and cannot lead to a recurrence.

WORK

For women who worked outside the home before treatment, returning to work is part of reestablishing a normal routine. Some women work full-time right away; others work part-time for a while before returning to a full-time schedule. Employers are usually willing to let a woman take time off for treatment (such as radiation therapy) or follow-up visits. Coworkers may be curious about a woman's absence and have questions about her treatment. Sharing information about the disease with coworkers can help ease the transition back to work.

ॐ

Resources for Breast Cancer Patients

American Cancer Society
1-800-ACS-2345
National Office
1599 Clifton Road, NE
Atlanta, Georgia 30329
http://www.cancer.org

The American Cancer Society is a voluntary national organization that supports research, conducts educational programs, and offers many services for patients and their families. The Reach to Recovery program is a rehabilitation program for women with breast cancer run by volunteers who have been treated for breast cancer. The trained volunteers provide assistance in meeting physical and psychological needs as well as practicalities of daily living. This service is offered free of charge. Information about services and activities in local areas can be obtained by calling or writing the national headquarters.

American Institute for Cancer Research
1-800-843-8114
1759 R St. NW
Washington D.C. 20009
http://www.aicr.org

The American Institute for Cancer Research focuses on the areas of diet and nutrition as they relate to the prevention and treatment of cancer. It is a leading source for educational programs for cancer prevention.

American Medical Association
1-800-621-8335
515 North State St.
Chicago, IL 60610
http://www.ama-assn.org

The American Medical Association is committed to providing timely information on matters important to the health of

America. Its website supplies information about breast cancer warning signs, mammograms and self-exams. It also contains search engines to locate doctors and hospitals in particular specialty areas and geographic locations.

American Medical Women's Association
1-703-838-0500
801 N. Fairfax St., Suite 400
Alexandria, VA 22314
http://www.amwa-doc.org

The American Medical Women's Association functions at the local, national, and international level to improve women's health. Their website contains information on breast cancer education, publications, and more.

Cancer Information Service
1-800-4-CANCER (M to F 9:00 am to 4:30 pm)
NCI Public Inquiries Office
6116 – Executive Blvd
MSC 8322, Room 3036A
Bethesda, MD 20892-8322
http://cis.nci.nih.gov

The Cancer Information Service, a program of the National Cancer Institute, provides a nationwide information and referral service, answering questions and mailing free information about treatment, support services, medical facilities, and more. The NCI website provides extensive information about treatment, clinical trials, statistics, and resources.

International Union Against Cancer
011-41-22-809-1811
3 rue du Conseil General
1205 Geneva, Switzerland
http://www.uicc.ch

The goals of the International Union Against Cancer are to advance scientific and medical knowledge in research, diagnosis, treatment, and prevention of cancer. Particular emphasis is placed on education. The website contains cancer news, press releases, publications, and links to other cancer resources.

Living Beyond Breast Cancer
1-888-753-LBBC
10 E. Athens Ave., Suite 204
Ardmore, PA 19003
http://www.lbbc.org

Living Beyond Breast Cancer is a non-profit educational organization committed to empowering all women affected by breast cancer to live as long as possible with the best quality of life. Programs include a quarterly educational newsletter, outreach to medically underserved women, and the Survivor's Helpline. The website provides educational materials, announcement of events, news, and links to other cancer resources.

National Coalition for Cancer Survivorship
1-877-NCCS YES
1010 Wayne Ave., Suite 770
Silver Spring, MD 20910-5600
http://www.canceradvocacy.org

The National Coalition for Cancer Survivorship raises awareness about cancer survivorship through its quarterly newsletter and other publications, conducts public education activities in an effort to eliminate the stigma of cancer, and offers advocacy for the insurance, employment, and legal rights of people with cancer. The coalition also serves as a facilitator of networking among cancer programs, offers information referrals, and promotes peer and professional support services. On a national level, NCCS provides public policy leadership on legislative, regulatory, and financing matters and promotes responsible advocacy among national cancer organizations.

Resources continued

Susan G. Komen Breast Cancer Foundation
1-800-IM-AWARE
5005 LBJ Freeway, Suite 250
Dallas, Texas 75244
http://www.komen.org

The Susan G. Komen Breast Cancer Foundation is a national organization that supports breast cancer research, education, screening, and treatment. Women may call the toll-free number to speak with a counselor about breast cancer screening, treatment options, and post-treatment support groups. The website provides news, links to other cancer resources, and live on-line chat groups with breast cancer experts.

Y-ME National Organization for Breast Cancer
1-800-221-2141
212 W. Van Buren, Suite 1000
Chicago, IL 60607-3908
http://www.y-me.org

The Y-ME National Organization for Breast Cancer offers information on treatment options and support groups. It has a 24-hour toll-free national hotline staffed by trained counselors and volunteers who have experienced breast cancer.

৯

Appendix: Breast Self-Examination

You should do breast self-examination (BSE) once a month to become familiar with the usual appearance and feel of your breasts. The best time to do BSE is 2 to 3 days after completion of your period, when your breasts are less swollen and tender. If you are postmenopausal, pick a day of the month that is easy to remember, such as the first day of the month or your birthday.

Most women have some lumps in their breasts. Doing BSE regularly will help you become familiar with the normal feel of your breasts. The important thing in BSE is to look and feel for changes. Figure 23 shows signs of possible breast cancer. The most

FIGURE 23

Signs of Possible Breast Cancer

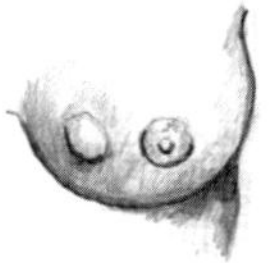

Lump
Usually single, firm, and most often painless

Inverted nipple
In a previously normal breast

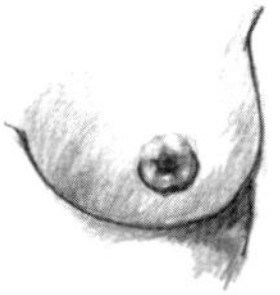

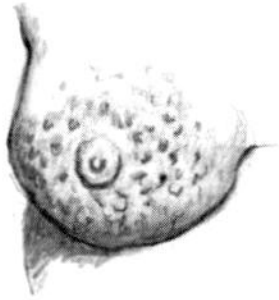

Change in skin's appearance
Portion of the skin on the breast has the appearance of an orange peel, sometimes accompanied by swelling

Superficial veins
Skin surface veins on one breast become more prominent than the other

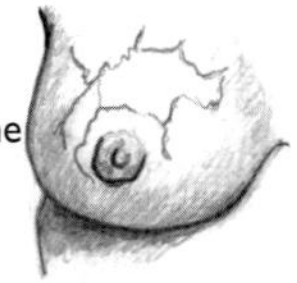

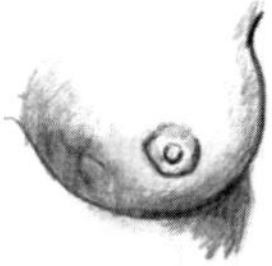

Skin dimpling
Depression occurring in a localized area of the breast surface

Myth

If I detected a lump in
my breast, it means
I have breast cancer.

Fact

Most lumps detected by
women on self-examination
are not cancer. If you detect
a lump or change in your
breast, it is important to
report this to your doctor
right away so that he or
she may examine you
and determine whether
further tests are needed.

common sign of breast cancer is a lump or thickness
that persists. Other signs to look for include swelling,
puckering, dimpling, redness, or soreness of the skin,
or a nipple that changes shape, becomes crusty, or
becomes inverted (drawn inward). Some women
have naturally inverted nipples. Most changes do not
mean that cancer is present. However, any change
should be fully evaluated by a doctor or nurse.

The Step-By-Step Guide on pages 51 to 54 will assist
you in performing breast self-examination. Begin by
looking at your breasts. Stand in front of a mirror with
your arms at your sides (Figure 24). Is the shape of the
breasts even without visible swelling or distortion? Are
both breasts their usual size, shape, and color? Is there
dimpling or puckering of the skin? Has the nipple of
either breast changed position? As you do the next two
steps, look for changes in the shape or contour of your
breasts. First, place your hands behind your head and
gently press them forward (Figure 25). Next, place your
hands on your hips and bend your shoulders and elbows
forward (Figure 26). Gently compress each nipple between
your fingers to check for discharge (Figure 27).

Next, feel your breasts. This can best be done while
you are bathing, when your skin is wet and soapy. Also,
feel the collarbone area and the axilla (armpit) on each
side (Figure 28). Next, support the left breast with the
left hand. Use the fingers of the right hand to compress
the breast, feeling for lumps or changes from the previous
month's exam. After feeling the entire breast, change
hands and repeat the process on the opposite side.

To complete the exam, lie down and carefully feel
each breast with the pads of the fingers of the opposite
hand (Figures 29 and 30). Examine the breast beginning at the edge of the nipple, feeling outward over the
entire breast mound. Use firm, smooth pressure so you
can feel the tissue beneath the skin. Be sure to press
underneath the nipple, feeling for firm nodules.

It is important to cover the entire breast. The best
way to do this is to follow a pattern. Some women
begin at the nipple and move around the breast in
larger and larger circles until they reach the outer edge
of the breast (Figure 31). Other women move their

fingers up and down imaginary vertical lines, gradually moving from one side of the breast to the other. Some women mentally divide the breast into wedges. They begin at the outer edge of a wedge and feel in toward the nipple, and then they move to the next wedge, repeating the process until the whole breast is covered.

Find a pattern that works for you and use it consistently. By being consistent, you will be more likely to notice any new lump or change in your breast.

If you have had surgical treatment for breast cancer, continue monthly BSE in addition to tests and exams done by your doctor or nurse. Some women are reluctant to examine themselves after surgery because they are afraid of finding a recurrence or new cancer. This may be a good opportunity to involve a spouse or partner in the healing process. A spouse or partner has strong motivation to help monitor the health of a loved one and will therefore be willing to offer encouragement, support, and reassurance.

When you do BSE after breast surgery, follow the steps outlined earlier in this chapter to examine the untreated breast. If you have had a segmental mastectomy, it is normal for the treated breast to feel firm and have a slightly altered contour, especially if you have had radiation therapy. It is important to become familiar with the normal look and feel of the treated breast so you will be able to notice any changes. When you examine the treated breast, pay close attention to the incision area, gently feeling for new nodules or other changes. If the entire breast was removed, the area where cancer is most likely to recur is beneath the skin on the chest wall. Therefore, this area should be examined closely each month. Carefully run the pads of the fingers of the opposite hand over the incision area, feeling for lumps or tiny nodules. Look at the scar for signs of redness, rash, or irritation.

Remember to perform your breast self-examination once a month. Follow the guidelines mentioned earlier in selecting a date to do your breast self-examination, that is 2 to 3 days after completion of your period, or a set day of the month that is easy to remember if you are postmenopausal (Figure 32).

I did my breast self-examination only because it was Breast Cancer Awareness Month. When I found the lump, I was shocked and afraid. After seeing my doctor for a clinical breast exam, I was so relieved to learn the lump was not cause for concern. Now I perform breast self-examination every month.

ৡ

Step-By-Step Guide

STEP 1

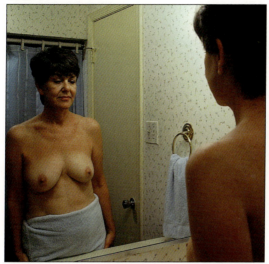

FIGURE 24

Visual Inspection of Breasts

STEP 2

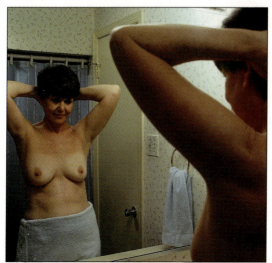

FIGURE 25

Arms Raised and Flexed

STEP 3

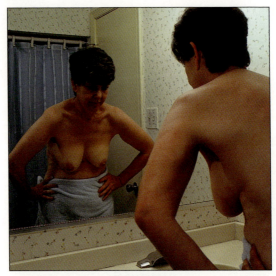

FIGURE 26
Arms Pressing Hips

STEP 4

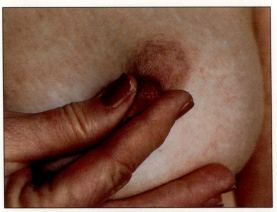

FIGURE 27
Check for Discharge

STEP 5

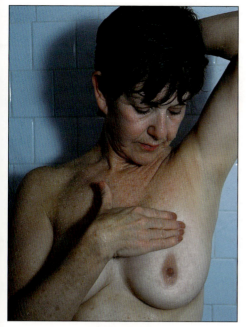

FIGURE 28

Feeling Breasts and Armpits While Standing

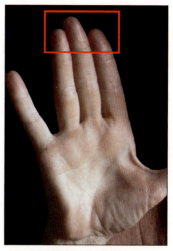

FIGURE 29

Use the Pads of Your Fingers

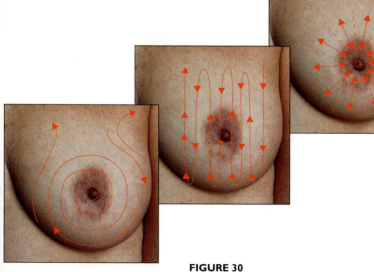

FIGURE 30

Patterns of Breast Self-Examination

STEP 6

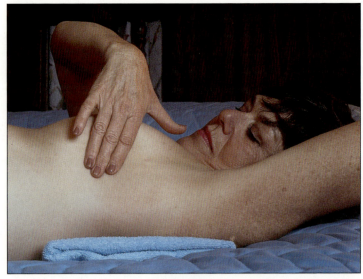

FIGURE 31
Feeling Breasts and Armpits While Lying Down

STEP 7
Repeat Step 5

STEP 8

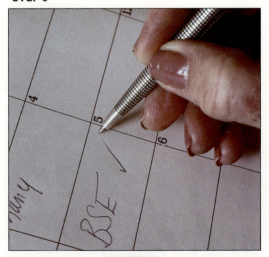

FIGURE 32
Breast Self-Examination Should be Performed Once a Month

Glossary

Adjuvant Therapy: Treatment given in addition to surgery, such as radiation therapy, chemotherapy, or hormonal therapy.

Antiestrogen Drugs: Drugs used in hormonal therapy. These agents block the effects of estrogen, a hormone that promotes the growth of some breast cancers.

Areola: The circular area around the nipple on the breast. The areola is typically darker than the rest of the breast.

Axilla: The armpit.

Axillary Lymph Nodes: The lymph nodes in the armpit.

Axillary Lymph Node Dissection: Surgery to remove some of the lymph nodes from the armpit.

Benign: Not cancerous.

Biopsy: A procedure in which a piece of tissue is removed and examined under a microscope.

Breast-Conserving Therapy: Treatment for breast cancer in which the breast is preserved. Breast-conserving therapy usually consists of segmental mastectomy and radiation therapy. Axillary lymph node dissection also may be done.

Breast Self-Examination: Examination of one's own breasts for changes. Any changes detected should be brought to the attention of a doctor or nurse.

Calcifications: Calcium deposits in the breast. Calcifications can be benign or malignant.

Cancer: The name given to a large group of diseases in which abnormal cells divide without control.

Central Venous Catheter: A flexible tube inserted into a large vein for the purpose of giving drugs or fluids. One end of the tube remains outside the body.

Chemotherapy: Treatment using cancer-fighting drugs.

Chemoprevention: Long-term treatment with an antiestrogen drug to reduce the occurrence of breast cancer in high-risk women.

Core Biopsy: Removal of a piece of tissue using a needle. The tissue is examined under a microscope to see if cancer cells are present. The patient is given a local anesthetic before a core biopsy is performed.

CT Scan: An abbreviation for "computed tomography scan," a type of scan in which X-rays are used to create cross-sectional pictures of the body.

Cyst: A fluid-filled sac.

Delayed Reconstruction: Reconstructive surgery done months or years after modified radical or total mastectomy.

Digital Mammography: A type of mammography in which images are preserved in electronic computer files rather than on film.

Drains: Devices used to remove fluid that collects at a surgery site. Drains are usually left in place for a short period after surgery. The drains used after breast surgery are usually made of tubing and suction bottles.

Ductal Carcinoma: Name given to any type of cancer that arises in the ducts of the breast.

Ducts: The channels in the breast that carry milk to the nipple.

Estrogen Receptor Assay: A test done on tumor tissue to find out if a tumor is sensitive to estrogen. The results of this test help determine whether hormonal therapy may be effective. Also called an estrogen receptor test or ER test.

Excisional Biopsy: Surgery to remove a tumor or mass. The tumor or mass is cut into thin sections that are studied under a microscope to see if cancer cells are present.

Fat Necrosis: Fat degeneration resulting in the development of hard, solid lumps in the breast. Fat necrosis is often the result of a blow to the breast.

Fibroadenoma: A benign tumor composed of fibrous tissue.

Fibrocystic Breast Disease: A term used to describe various benign breast conditions.

Fine-Needle Aspiration (FNA): A type of biopsy in which cells are removed from a lump using a needle and syringe. The cells are studied under a microscope to see if cancer cells are present.

Hormonal Therapy: Treatment using drugs to block the effect of certain hormones and thus slow tumor growth.

Hyperplasia: A condition in which there is an abnormal increase in the number of cells in a tissue.

Immediate Reconstruction: Reconstructive surgery done at the same time as modified radical or total mastectomy.

Implant: An artificial device sometimes used in reconstructive surgery to create a breast shape. Implants are silicone bags filled with saline or silicone gel.

Invasive: Growing into and destroying healthy tissue. Tumors can be either invasive or noninvasive.

Lobular Carcinoma: Name given to any type of cancer that arises in the lobules of the breast.

Lobules: Milk-producing glands within the breast.